JOSEPH FIORE JR

Healthy Self

The Easiest Way to Get Healthy, Lose Weight and Transform Yourself in 30 Days

This book was professionally typeset on Reedsy.
Find out more at reedsy.com

Contents

Introduction

I am so excited to be writing this book and sharing these tactics for you to reach your health and physical potential over the next 30 days. This book is an easy step by step guide to improve your health in every way from weight loss to better sleep and feeling better overall. These are the very tips and tricks I used everyday to lose over 20 pounds in the last year and keep it all off, all the while increasing my work productivity, fitness capacity, and even lab results. The goal of this book is to give you these simple, affordable, daily tasks to take full control of your health.

A little about myself, my name is Joe Fiore and I am a physical therapist with 20+ years of experience in practice and a background in strength and conditioning. I have helped thousands of patients regain function through lifestyle changes and exercise. I have found recently that the ideas and habits outlined in this book have provided the best short term results that turn into long term success for myself and hundreds of patients in my clinic. I truly have a passion for helping others not only recover from injury, but maximize their health for the long haul. I have seen this exact program work time after time from the young athlete trying to enhance performance, to the elderly grandmother taking care of her family. I hope that you can follow through and reach your potential.

The current state of American health is at best abysmal. Current estimates of obesity include 42% of adults and 19% of children. Not only is obesity on the rise, but extreme obesity is also climbing at an alarming rate rising from almost 0% in 1970 to almost 9% in 2017-

18. Obesity is directly linked to multiple health issues including: Type 2 Diabetes and Pre-Diabetes, dyslipidemia (out of whack cholesterol, triglycerides, inflammation), heart disease, sleep disorders, cognitive dysfunctions, liver disease, and cancer to name a few. Obesity has been shown to be more complex than simply eating too much and not moving enough. There are multiple systems at play including hormonal changes, mitochondrial functions, circadian rhythms to give you an idea. This guide book aims to target each of these arms of obesity to help you achieve your health goals.

Heart disease is still a leading cause of death here in the United States. According to the CDC one person dies every 33 seconds from heart disease and 1 in 5 deaths are related to heart disease. Coronary Artery Disease is the most common form of heart disease and affects about 1 in 20 adults over the age of 20. Heart disease is not just a concern for the elderly. About 1 in 5 deaths are in people under the age of 65. Heart attacks are also one of the leading causes of death. Every 40 seconds someone in the US suffers a heart attack. Again, there are many factors that affect someone's risk for heart disease, and the tips and tricks offered here are not cures, but can help cut down the risk you may have by improving your overall health and wellness.

Chronic disease can be defined as conditions that last over a year and require medical care or limit activities of daily living or both. Common chronic diseases include: Diabetes, some cancers, auto-immune diseases, osteoporosis, and dementias of all kinds. Some causes of chronic disease are linked directly to lifestyle choices. Smoking, excessive alcohol intake, lack of movement, poor nutrition, lack of vitamins and minerals, circadian mismatches can all lead to the advancement of chronic diseases.

In this book, I am going to share with you some simple daily actions that can have a true effect on all of the above lifestyle risk factors for these health pitfalls. We are going to cover how to use fasting, grounding, sunlight, hot and cold exposure, and exercise as tools to shed weight, improve metabolism, reset circadian rhythms and help hormonal balances. If you can commit to following the daily plan laid out for you, I have no doubt that you will feel and act like a different human. I want to strongly encourage you to work with your physician while on this journey. Be sure to keep track of all of your labs, weight, subjective feeling, sleep, etc in order to see the difference in your health. I have no doubt that you will be doing things that you may never have thought possible. I see it everyday in the clinic, people just like you doing amazing things they never thought possible.

Let me share a couple of quick stories. The first is Adam, a young man and wrestler that I had the privilege of coaching for some time. When his senior year rolled around, he decided it would be best to drop from the 285 pound weight class to the 220 pound weight class. Now, when we started, he weighed right around 280 pounds during football season. We started his weight cut in October, and the first week of January he made the weight at 220. He went on to finish third in the state that year in wrestling. In addition to making his weight, we noticed that his chronic eczema had cleared up substantially by following the health hacks outlined in this book.

A more recent example is a patient we will call Karen. Karen came to me with chronic pain all over her body, and was weighing well over 300 pounds. She had trouble walking, sitting and standing from a chair, traveling, doing almost anything. I was able to set her up with just a couple of items from this book, and she still was able to lose over 60 pounds. I had not seen her in a couple of years until just very recently for a different injury, and the weight has been kept off. I bet she has continued to lose weight, and just hasn't kept track! Better yet, most of her pain has gone away and she is back to living her life and enjoying her hobbies once again.

Over the next five chapters, we will dive a little deeper into each discipline to reach your potential. This book is designed to be a guide; I could write an entire book of its own on each topic. I want this book to be an action plan for your success. We will look into the research of fasting, grounding, sunlight, hot and cold exposure, and exercise. We will form a daily ritual for you to follow in order to maximize your results. Now, every individual has their own biology, needs, levels of dysfunction, environment, genetic factors, etc. It will be imperative that some common sense be followed and tweaked along the way. This is not a cookie cutter, one size fits all type of situation, but I am convinced that by following these tenets to the best of your ability you will yield tremendous health benefits for years to come.

1

Chapter 1 Fasting

The use of fasting as medicine dates back to at least the Ancient Greeks and Hippocrates, who would instruct patients of his to abstain from food if demonstrating certain ailments. Religious fasting dates back thousands of years as well. From pagan ceremonies to all forms of current religious practices, and across all faiths, fasting plays a role in the celebration of holidays and sacred teachings. Fasting began to be studied in a more scientific way starting in the 19th century. Throughout the 19th and 20th centuries, fasting was regularly used in the medical community to treat certain illnesses. Throughout that time, different forms of fasting started to emerge. Long duration, sometimes up to a month, was thought to cure many ailments of the time. Modified fasting became common where a patient was allowed a certain number of calories per day. Intermittent fasting has recently become popular again over the last decade.

We will focus on the current state of fasting to make your success as easy as possible. Now, again, you will be able to tweak this program to fit your individual needs, and find what works best for your individual situation.

We will begin with intermittent fasting (IF). What is IF? How does IF work? Let's dive in. The most important thing to know about IF is that success is less about *what* you eat, and more about *when* you eat. When we are in a period of fasting, with no food or energy coming in, the body will burn the sugar that is available to keep the systems online. The body can learn to switch between energy sources. The common energy sources needed are sugar and carbohydrates, and fat. These energy sources come from the food we eat. If we are not active enough during the day, we will not burn off the food we consume, and that can lead to storing excess fat, thus leading to obesity. The body will default to burning sugar first, as it is easiest to convert to energy for the body. Once all of the sugar in the system is gone, the body will then turn to the fat stores for energy. This is where IF can make a huge difference.

Simply put, by increasing the amount of time between meals, the body has more opportunity to burn fat for energy. Most Americans eat three meals a day, plus snacks. This set up continually feeds the body new energy and sugar sources, and the body will never get to the fat stores. Additionally, most Americans are not active enough during the day to use up all of the sugar. If that sugar is not used readily, it will be stored as fat. We will use IF to force the body to burn fat between feedings and lower your body weight.

In addition to losing weight, there are other documented benefits to IF. Studies have shown that IF can not only help with obesity but also prevent Type 2 Diabetes, heart disease, bowel disorders, and cognitive dysfunction. IF has been shown to boost memory, improve blood pressure, heart rate, reduce blood glucose levels (important to prevent type 2 diabetes), even helping with tissue recovery after injury or surgery.

Is it safe? For most of the population, IF is completely safe, however, precautions should be taken, and monitoring from a physician is indicated if you have the following: if you are a child under 18, if you are pregnant or nursing, people with Type 1 diabetes, and those with a history of eating disorders. If you do not fall into one of the above categories, feel free to jump right in. IF does not have to be temporary, in fact some of my most successful clients long term have just stayed on an IF program as their normal day to day life. It is important to note that some people will have different experiences on IF, and need to speak to a doctor if feeling headaches, nausea or other symptoms that occur.

OK, now you have decided to start. What does IF look like? Simple. There are a couple of different plans that I have seen work time and time again. The first, and maybe the most common, is a daily fast. All you have to do is pick an 8 hour window to eat all of your meals within. Once that 8 hour window closes, you abstain from food. For example, I used to eat between 11 am and 7 pm. That 8 hour eating window worked well with my lifestyle. I could get to work, eat lunch around 11 am, have another meal once home, and supper with my wife and children. Once 7 pm rolled around, I knew I was done eating for the day. I lived this lifestyle for many years. Any 8 hour window will work; you will have to find what works best, and is the easiest to follow. For some, 7 am to 3 pm is best, or noon to 8 pm. Could be 9 am to 5 pm, any 8 hour window will drive the changes you are looking for.

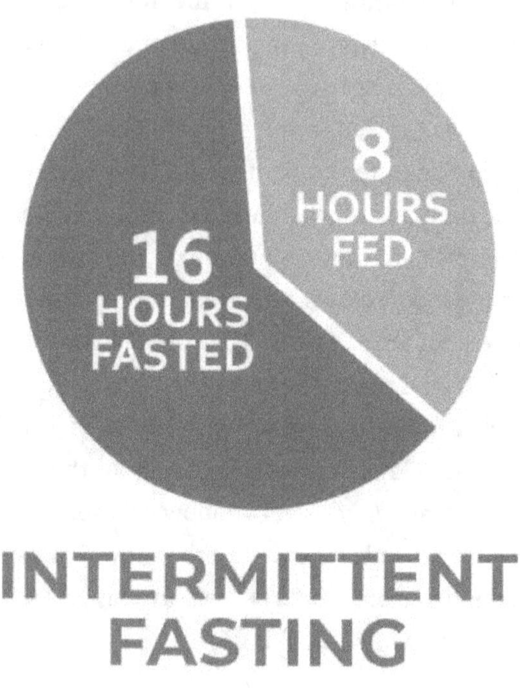

16:8 Intermittent Fasting

Another option is what is called a 5/2 plan. This strategy involves eating in your normal pattern over five days of the week, then limiting yourself to one small meal a day for two days. For example, Monday and Friday you will only eat one small meal a day, and the rest of the week will be normal. On Monday and Friday in the example, you would only eat one meal, consisting of about 500-600 calories. The days of the week do not matter, but the ratio does. You will have to be disciplined to eat only one meal a day while in the 2 day fasting period. The fasting days can be split up throughout the week whenever is best for you, but should not be two consecutive days.

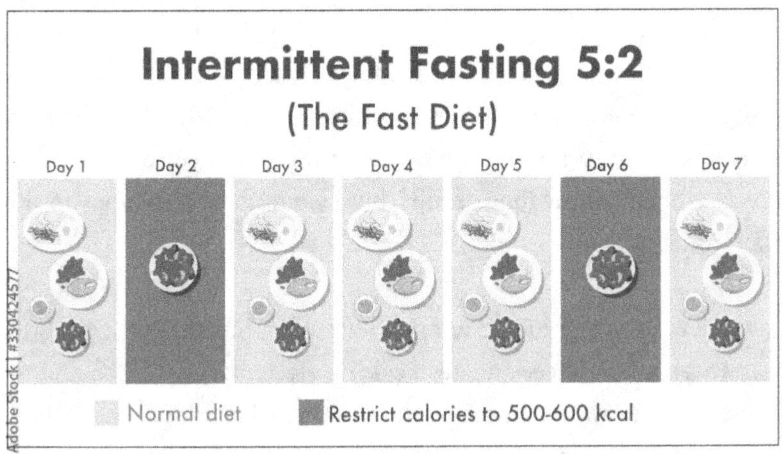

5:2 Intermittent Fasting

A third, and final option for this book, is Circadian fasting. What does that mean? Circadian fasting means planning and eating all of your meals within daylight. Circadian rhythm is the natural changes in the body that occur over a 24 hour period of time. It is our internal clock that tells us when to wake, when to sleep, when to rest, when to be active. It is the natural occurring blueprint for our bodies to follow on a daily basis. There is promising research on the impact that sunlight can have on health, and on the contrary, how artificial light can throw off our Circadian rhythm and lead to health issues. This option of only eating during daylight may have profound effects on health and wellness beyond what IF can do. This is personally the fasting program I use currently. I have tried all three IF programs listed, and prefer the

Circadian Fasting program for my health goals.

What should I eat? This is a topic worthy of an entire book to itself. I will encourage you to eat real food, not any of the processed junk that populates so much of the American diet. Stick to meats (unless you are vegan, vegetarian, etc), veggies, fruit, nuts. I will suggest avoiding sugary drinks, candy, gluten (if allergic), juices, soda. Strive for clean foods, fresh meat, dairy (unless you are allergic), fresh fruit, fresh veggies. The nice thing about the IF program is that you can still enjoy choices from all of the food groups, but I would caution anyone to stay away from junk food.

What about during the fast? Won't I get hungry? Initially maybe. Stick with water, tea, coffee, and zero calorie electrolytes. Coffee and tea offer appetite suppressing benefits as well as taking up space as liquid in the stomach. Zero calorie electrolyte drinks or packets are essential in order to function at the highest level. Electrolyte packets should contain sodium, potassium, magnesium to start.

   Lastly, a quick word of caution. The body may take a week or two to adjust to IF. It is quite possible and likely that you will experience an initial dip in energy, feel tired, hungry or cranky. This is normal, and most likely from a withdrawal period as your body changes. During that time, focus on the benefits you will start to reap. It is not unusual for clients to lose 7-10 pounds in that first week or two, so focus on the positive!!!

2

Chapter 2 Grounding

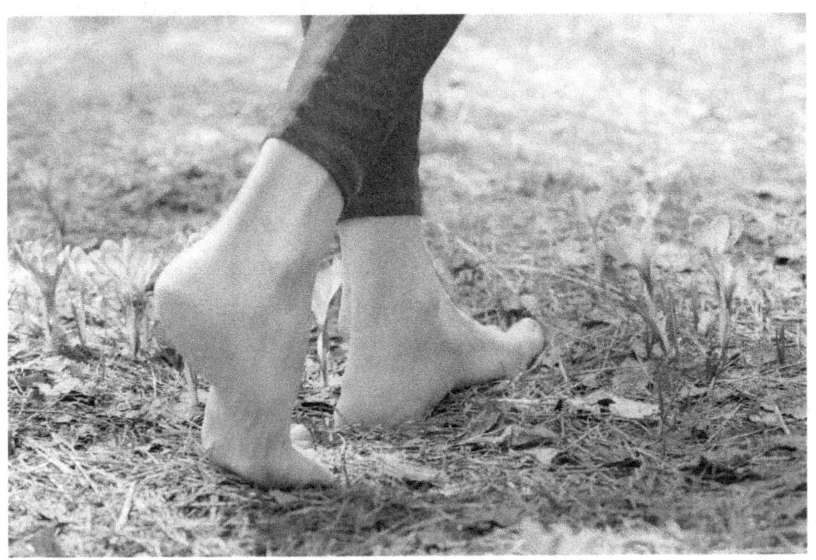

Barefoot Grounding

What the heck is Grounding? Simply put, it is standing with your bare skin in contact with the earth. Standing barefoot in the grass, digging up the dirt in a garden, touching a live tree or any product that is directly placed into the earth.

We, as humans, are electrically charged beings, and so is the Earth. We will have to dive into some physics here, but bear with me. Our bodies are made up of batteries, and occasionally need to be recharged. One of the best ways to recharge is to simply make contact with the Earth. The Earth is also made up of batteries, and can share energy with us to bring us back to balance. The most important part of our batteries are particles called electrons (this is as complex as the physics will get). We can share electrons with our environment. We naturally lose electrons throughout our daily lives and that can lead to issues like decreased energy, poor sleep, increased inflammation. Some experts believe that by grounding, we can receive fresh electrons from the Earth to replace the ones lost during the day.

How does it work? Experts believe that the sharing of electrons is just a part of nature. The human body is capable of exchanging electrons and absorbing them into the body. It is thought that this phenomenon can make changes in the body to improve health. There is a correlation over time of human interaction with the earth decreasing, and chronic illness increasing. Now, this is not to say that the lack of current grounding across humans is the single cause of all of our ailments. Some experts believe, though, that some of today's health crisis arises when we stopped spending time outside with our bodies in direct contact with the surface of the Earth. When we absorb these electrons from the Earth, they act as antioxidants and neutralize damaging compounds in the body to ensure a healthy outcome.

Grounding has been shown to improve sleep, help heal wounds, and decrease inflammation throughout the body. Studies have shown that the simple act of grounding can decrease inflammatory markers in the body, thus reducing certain ailments related to inflammation. The researchers in that study were able to find less inflammatory molecules in the tissues of people that grounded regularly versus those that did not. Another study looked at the difference in blood thickness between groups of people using a grounding mat for yoga versus those that did not. Again, the researchers found that those who grounded for an hour had less blood thickness, and better blood flow. Increased blood viscosity is linked to certain disease processes like hypertension, diabetes, and heart disease. Still another study confirmed that grounding results in better and deeper sleep, especially in the restorative phase of sleep. Maybe that is why people feel so much better during and after a beach vacation!!

How do I do it? Simple. Get outside and get your feet in the dirt or grass. This is something that can be done just about anywhere and at any time. Try to start with 5-10 minutes per day, then increase as much as you can. I routinely spend 30 plus minutes a day in my yard barefoot! If the idea of being barefoot is too much, try gardening for 5-10 minutes per day, or leaning on a tree with your palms on the tree. If that is too much for you, wearing leather soled shoes in the grass, or even on concrete will do the trick. Of course, in this modern era, there are a number of grounding products on the market. I have not tried them, as I tend to be more old fashioned, but they include: mats, sheets, shoes, socks, rods and mattress pads.

3

Chapter 3 Sunlight

An absolute must for optimizing health and wellness is a plan to increase sunlight tolerance and exposure. Think about this for just a minute. What source of energy is responsible for all of the life on the planet? It is the sun. So just think, if the sun can power all of the natural occurring processes to sustain life, how can it be so bad for us?? I just do not see it that way. Now, anything taken to an extreme can be harmful, so use common sense. If you can build a healthy relationship with the sun, the health benefits are too plentiful to name in this short chapter. We will focus on a few of the big benefits to get the most out of your time in the sun!!

Think about your family members, past and present. When my grandfather was alive, and his generation was walking the earth, there was minimal obesity in adults and especially children. Almost all people in photos from the 1930's through the 1980's were thin, healthy looking and tan. That generation spent much more time outside than we currently do! When I think back to my childhood in the 1980's and 1990's growing up, we were outside all of the time. I was fortunate enough to grow up near a forest preserve outside of Chicago, IL, and that was our playground. All summer long specifically, we would leave the house after breakfast, play until lunch, head back out until dark. We did not need sunscreen, we did not play video games or watch TV all day. When I think about my own children, despite my efforts and encouragement, they spend more time inside than I ever did. Adults and children today are much more susceptible to illness and poor health at least in part due to lack of sun exposure.

Think about a typical day for you or a child you know. Wake up, maybe before sunrise, most likely not. Get into a car to go to school or work, still inside. Maybe walk from the parking lot to the school or office, so maybe up to 10 minutes outside if you have to park blocks away!! Spend the next 6-8 hours inside school or work, surrounded by artificial light everywhere, staring at screens all day. Get in the car and head home. If you are lucky, maybe the sun is still up while you prepare a meal and get ready for supper. Maybe you or the kids have a sport activity a few hours a week outside, that is it! Then it is TV and phone before bed. If we add up all of the minutes and seconds spent outside in a typical day it might equate to an average of one hour a day. We have got to do better. Now, again, I am not saying get outside tomorrow for ten hours, and come home burnt. That is not the goal. I will walk you through a strategy to build your tolerance in the sun, and all of the benefits the sun can offer.

Let's talk about the benefits of the sun. Again, this will be a quick overview. There are enough benefits from the sun to dedicate an entire book to them. We will focus on Vitamin D, antibacterial properties, reduced blood pressure, improved sleep, and supporting weight loss.

Vitamin D. One of the master hormones. Proper levels of Vitamin D are strongly correlated with overall greater health. People with higher Vitamin D levels get sick less often, have less chances of being obese, are at less risk for almost all cancers, have stronger bones and less risk of bone diseases, have less depression, and less dementia. The list goes on and on. The best way to boost Vitamin D is to be in the sun. Depending on skin tone, people will require different amounts of time in the sun. Pale skinned people can get benefits in as little as 10 minutes, whereas darker skinned people may need 20-30 minutes. Where you live also plays a role. Living closer to the equator requires less time in the sun, than living farther away from the equator. The key takeaway is to avoid sunburn at all cost.

The sun acts as a strong antibiotic. The sun is made up of many different types of light, and UV light kills many bacteria. In multiple studies, UV light kills many forms of bacteria that cause infection and allergies. Most of these bacteria are present in the dust inside of our homes. So, get outside, open some windows and get that sunlight and fresh air into your homes as much as possible!

Exposure to sunlight can lower blood pressure. In multiple studies, people who sat in the sun lowered their blood pressure. The theory is that the UV light acts on the blood vessels and dilates them, making them larger and blood flows with greater ease. When blood pressure is better controlled, there is less risk for heart disease and strokes! Wouldn't it be great to potentially not have to take medications, but just sit in the sun to lower blood pressure?

The sun helps with sleep. Sun exposure plays a large role in managing the natural circadian rhythm as discussed in an earlier chapter. Early morning sun can set the stage for falling asleep easier in the coming evening. Exposure to sunrise triggers the production and eventual release of the hormone melatonin. Melatonin is known as the sleep hormone. In order for your body to make this sleep hormone naturally, you need to see the morning sun preferably with the naked eye. That does not mean stare directly into the sun!! Just no sunglasses, and gaze at the horizon. It is truly as simple as that for a better night's sleep.

Sun exposure supports weight loss. Scientists are not exactly sure how, but people who spend more time outdoors in the sun have lower body mass indices. I am sure the sun regulates many hormonal and circadian clocks that help to regulate metabolism, but I am not a researcher! There are many theories tied to weight loss and weight management, but circadian rhythm is a vital player in obesity. If being out in the sun raises Vitamin D, improves sleep, prevents infections, among many other benefits, it only stands to reason that obesity can be decreased as well.

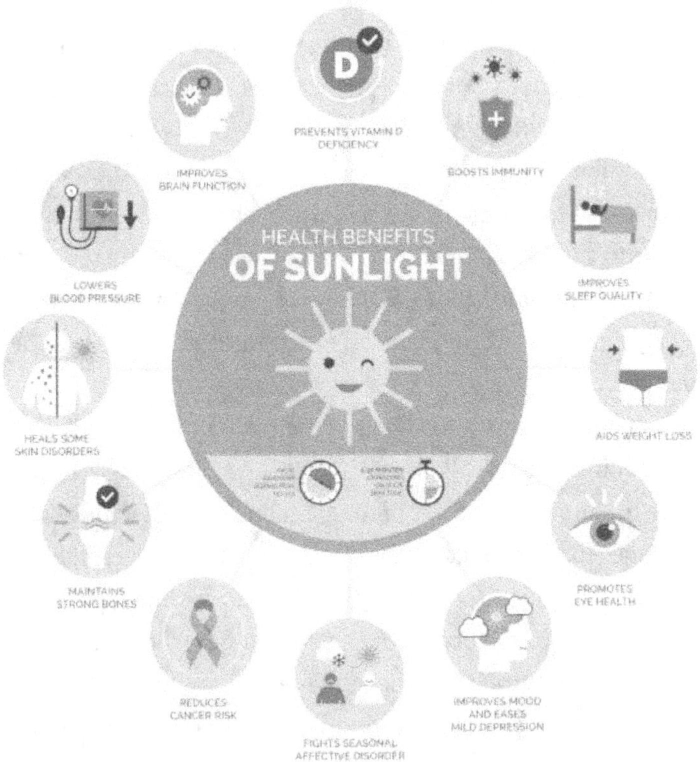

Benefits of Sunlight

How do I maximize the sun's benefits? The most important thing I think a person can do to drastically improve health and wellness is see the sunrise. I make sure I am outside as the sun is coming up everyday. Some days I will only have a few minutes, others maybe up to 30. I make sure I can see the horizon, and I do not wear sunglasses or sunscreen. The early morning sun is what is called full spectrum, meaning all types of light are present from infrared to ultraviolet in a magnificent, perfect balance. That early morning sun exposure will set the tone for your day, and get all of the hormonal and metabolic activities firing for your success. As the day progresses, I will keep trying to sneak out of the office for quick exposures to the sun. On my days off, I will try and spend more time in the sun. I happen to work in a physical therapy office with great big windows, and we will open the windows as often as possible to let the light in. I know that is not an option for all people. Another tip and trick is to drive with your windows down, even a crack, is enough to get sunlight into your eyes and on your skin. Once that early morning sun hits your eyes, the brain knows it is time to get the day started. The eyes are the gateway to the brain, and all of the internal clocks that need to be regulated.

Once you have gotten in the habit of seeing the sunrise daily, it is safe to start building what is called a solar callus. A solar callus is how I build tolerance to the sun, just like building a callus on your hands with hard work. It takes time and small increments of exposure. Again, I am not a fan of sunglasses or sunscreens, as that distorts the messaging from the skin and the eyes to the brain, and can affect how the brain interprets your circadian rhythm, hormonal and metabolic activity. I do not ever want to burn. When I started this journey a few years ago, I would only spend 5-10 minutes at a time in the sun. Then about every month, I would add 5-10 more minutes of sun bathing. Over time, I have built a tolerance where I can go hours in the sun even at peak times with no sunglasses or sunscreen without burning. But please, I implore you, to use common sense and avoid burning at all costs!! Work with your physician if needed to build a plan that is best for you.

You may be wondering why no sunglasses? The simple answer is that sunglasses alter the information going to the brain. The eyes communicate with the brain the time of the day it is, and how intense the sun is during the day. The first part, the time, keeps the brain on top of our circadian rhythm, and keeps our bodies in balance. Secondly, the eyes communicate the intensity of the sun, and the brain and other tissues will release melanin to protect the skin from the rays of the sun, resulting in a greater tan.

A brief discussion on artificial light. We are surrounded by artificial light most of the time. In order to achieve maximal health and wellness, we need to turn down the light at night. Research has found that artificial light at night is linked to increased risks of cancers, diabetes, heart disease, circadian rhythm disruption, sleep disorders, psychological problems just to name a few. The best thing one can do to minimize these risks is to turn off the lights at night completely. If that is not an option, here are some helpful strategies. I wear blue light blocking glasses after dark at night if I am working or watching TV. You can change the light bulb types in your house to incandescent if possible. Blackout curtains are a great option if you live in an urban area to decrease the exposure to street lamps, etc. Some of my clients have had success with sleep masks as well. Anything we can do to limit artificial light at night exposure will be great for your health!!

Summarizing the action plan for sunlight. Make sure to see the sunrise every morning, give yourself short and frequent exposures during the day, and turn off the lights at night! Commit to these habits and see the changes in your health dramatically improve in the next month!!

4

Chapter 4 Exercise

What can I say about exercise that has not already been poured over, studied and implemented? The benefits of exercise are exhaustive, and again, too big a scope for this book. I will try and cover the basics, and offer a simple plan to get you started on your exercise journey. The main health benefits of exercise we will focus on include controlling weight, fighting illness and disease, improving mood, and better sleep. These are the big rocks that come with exercise. Again, there are countless more benefits that can fill an entire book just about exercise.

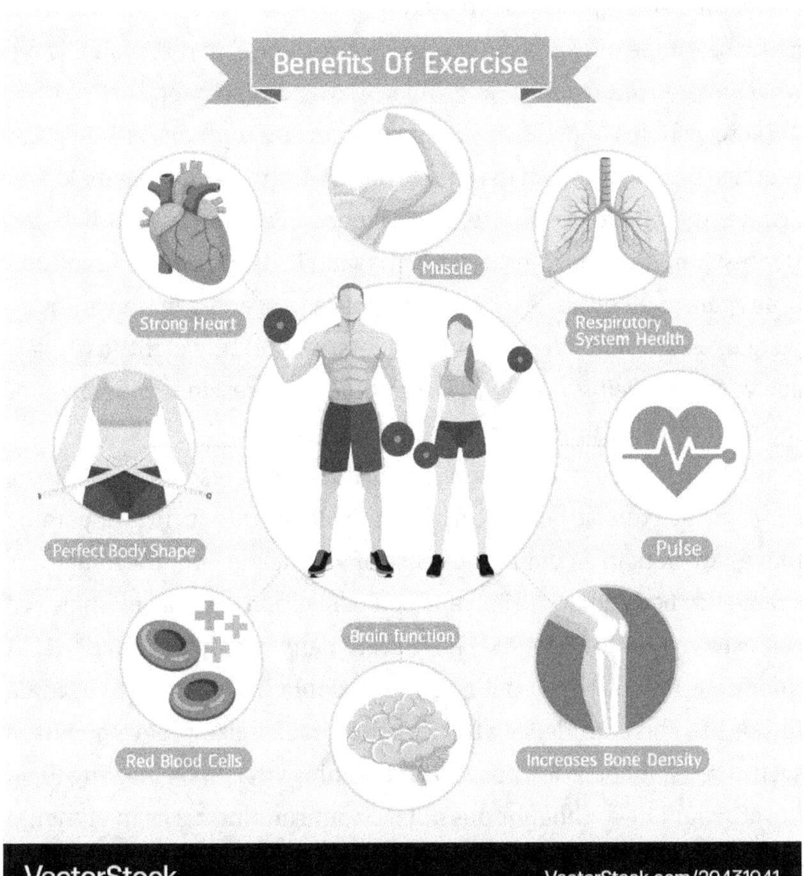

Exercise helps with weight control. Obesity and weight gain are quite complicated and encompass more than just calories in and calories out, but being active plays a large role in controlling how much weight one carries. The good news is that we do not have to put in hours and hours of training to get the weight control benefits of exercise. Staying active, and keeping the body lean can lead to all kinds of health benefits. Exercise needs to be a part of everyone's daily routine for health and wellness. My general rule of thumb is to break a sweat everyday. Some days my training is with some form of cardiovascular training, but could be weight training, yoga, or circuit training. Oftentimes, I get asked what is the best type of exercise? My answer is always, and I mean always, whatever you like the best, and will be most consistent at.

Exercise helps boost the immune system and fight disease. Regular exercise has been shown to reduce the risk for the following maladies: Stroke, metabolic syndrome, high blood pressure, Type 2 diabetes, Depression, Anxiety, Cancer, Arthritis, and Falls. I have seen time and time again as a Physical Therapist the power of exercise in transforming people. From reducing pain in patients, to seeing weight loss goals achieved, to seeing people blossom out of depression, the power of regular exercise cannot be overstated.

As alluded to above, exercise can even improve a person's mood. In the short term, exercise boosts certain brain chemicals such as dopamine that give a person an uplift and sense of well being. Over the long term, changes in body composition, and self perception can lead to improved self esteem and confidence. I have seen many examples of patients of mine that have stepped out of a life of doubt and anxiety to become full of life and confidence after starting an exercise program. I have seen dozens, if not more, people achieve things that upon meeting them never would have thought possible. From running races to climbing mountains, from competing in sports to playing with grandchildren, the power of exercise is profound for most!

Sleep, what does exercise do for sleep? Regular exercise helps the brain focus on regulating the internal clocks that keep us healthy. Any activity that will enhance the ability to fall asleep and stay asleep will have an immense effect on our overall health and wellness.

So, all of this sounds great, but how do I do it? Again, this book is designed to give you some step by step actions to get you going. The topic of exercise is too immense, and could be the source for multiple books. I want to focus on two types of exercise for you. The first is cardiovascular training. We will define cardiovascular training as anything gets your heart rate elevated. This could be walking, jogging, running, cycling, rowing, etc. This list can go on for just about a mile! I want you to focus on breaking a sweat everyday. Choose an activity that is enjoyable, repeatable, and safe. Experts recommend 150 to 300 minutes of moderate cardiovascular exercise a week. That is less than an hour a day at an easy to moderate pace. Some of you wont have that much time per day, so I will recommend shorter duration, more intense work for you. If you only have a few minutes, choose an activity that will challenge you more than an easy jog or walk. Try a TABATA class, spin class, jump rope, etc. Again, there are a million options out there to get your exercise in!!

The second form of exercise that is vital to great health and wellness is strength training. Strength training involves pushing your body against resistance to train the muscles. Strength training can be performed in various ways as well. I want you to focus on strength training 30-60 minutes up to three times a week. Strength training can take different forms, but must involve resistance at all times. Strength training can be body weight exercises like push-ups and pull-ups, can involve the use of free weights like dumbbells and kettle bells, or bands like you see in the therapy clinics. In the big scheme of things, the type of resistance is less important than the consistency of performing the exercises. I use all types of equipment in my own training and in the training of my patients and clients. There is no wrong way to exercise as long as you remain safe!!

A sample week of training can look like the following:

- Cardio training on Monday, Wednesday, Friday.
- Strength training on Tuesday, Thursday, Saturday.
- Rest day on Sunday. Sunday may also be a great day for the sauna or ice bath (see following chapter).

5

Chapter 5 HOT and COLD

The proper use of hot and cold exposure is an absolute cheat code to reach your potential. I have used the sauna and cold plunges in order to take my health and mental toughness to the next level. Not only does the sauna and cold plunge offer outstanding physical benefits, but the mental upsides are second to none. We will briefly describe the benefits of both the sauna and cold plunge, and how to implement each modality into your wellness routine.

Let us start with the heat. We will be discussing the use of saunas to improve health. There are typically two types of sauna available. The traditional sauna, set at 160 degrees Fahrenheit in most research settings, and the infrared sauna. The traditional sauna has been used for thousands of years, and uses dry heat produced by heating up stones. The typical sauna is set to 160 degrees Fahrenheit and the session lasts up to 20 minutes. Infrared (IR) saunas use light to produce the heat, and typically are not as hot as the traditional sauna, but may offer other benefits not seen by the traditional sauna. IR light has been shown to have significant health benefits separate from the heat produced. Saunas and heat exposure has been linked with lowering blood pressure, lowering risk for heart disease, preventing illness and possibly cognitive diseases.

How do I get these benefits? Most research suggests that at least one sauna session a week at 20 minutes is enough to increase your overall health. Most research suggests that sauna sessions greater than once a week continues to lower risk for the above mentioned ailments. The degree and frequency is really up to the person. I personally like to be in the sauna at least once a week for up to 20-30 minutes, more often when time allows. It has taken me a few years of regular visits to the sauna in order to build that tolerance though. When starting out, make sure to listen to your body and do not ignore signs of dehydration. Signs of dehydration include:

- Thirst
- Dry or sticky mouth
- Not peeing very much
- Dark yellow pee
- Dry, cool skin
- Headache
- Muscle cramps
- Confusion

The risks of sauna, though minimal, do exist. Of the people who suffer injury from saunas, most have alcohol involved. On sauna day, it is extremely important to avoid alcohol at all costs, and stay hydrated. There are some health conditions which make the sauna unsafe. If you have any of the following conditions, I would recommend staying out of the sauna unless cleared by your physician: Aortic valve stenosis, chest pain, heart attack. Take precaution and get clearance from a physician if you are over 65, pregnant, or have a seizure disorder. Children under the age of seven are recommended to stay out of the sauna as well.

Cold plunging has become all of the rage over the last few years, and for good reason. I have been experimenting on myself with cold exposure for about seven years now. Getting comfortable with the unique discomfort of the cold has been a truly enlightening experience for me, and the clients that have taken the journey with me. I am always amazed at the outcome that a client, or even my sons have had with the ice bath. Let us find out what is so great about cold exposure, and how to implement these techniques into your optimal health routine.

I will do my best to summarize the numerous benefits of cold plunging, as the topic deserves an entire book unto itself! In general, the ice bath and cold exposure has been shown to drive metabolic changes, restore hormonal balances, decrease inflammation, reduce soreness from training, and improve the immune system. The use of cold exposure has been shown to change the type of fat in our bodies. Yes, there are two types of fat, brown fat and white fat. Brown fat is much healthier, packed with mitochondria and much more metabolically active. White fat is much more inert, and may be responsible for many of the inflammatory troubles some people encounter. The great thing about cold exposure, is the body can turn white fat into brown fat, thus helping someone lose weight and decrease inflammation!

How do I start? Slowly. Getting into the cold is not easy, and precautions must be taken. The temperature of the water does not need to be below 50 degrees Fahrenheit. I know there are folks out there that can tolerate sub 40 degree water, but the research is pretty clear. 50 degrees will give you all of the benefits without the risk of injury. There are a number of ways to get started. One popular way is face dunking. Fill a large bowl with ice and water, shooting for 50-55 degrees Fahrenheit, and place your entire face in the bowl. Hold your face under for up to 30 seconds. You can repeat this procedure a few times and be done. Another option is cold showers. Every morning, regardless if I have taken an ice bath that day or not, I finish with a cold shower. For the beginner, start your shower warm, and then turn the water temperature as cold as you can stand for 10, 15 seconds. Then, progress to 30 seconds and finally a full minute. If you have access to an actual cold plunge, try and get neck deep for 1-3 minutes. Once you can control your breathing, and you will start to get comfortable with ice baths, work your way up to 5 minutes or so. I do not think staying in an ice bath beyond 10 minutes is necessary at all. If none of this sounds doable for you, try driving with your windows down in winter for short distances (less than 20 minutes) or walking through the parking lot without a jacket. Do not, and I repeat, do not risk hypothermia for any potential benefits.

The use of cold exposure is one of the hardest things a person can do, but those who overcome the fear and discomfort become much more resilient, happier, and healthier. When you enter that cold water, know that you will hyperventilate some. Make sure to focus on breathing, and slow it down. I made a habit of counting while breathing in and out, trying to get to four or five while breathing. Once calm, I would use my time on the ice to pray, think, meditate, and make my daily affirmations. I would typically perform my ice baths in the morning, mostly because of my schedule.

6

Chapter 6 Putting it all together

At this point, you might be asking how the heck do I do all of this? Let me help you. Let me share my typical day, and then help you come up with a health and wellness schedule. It will be up to you to make your health a priority. Now, let me tell you, I see patients day in and day out that only wish they would have made health a bigger priority in life. I have patients that come in everyday with bodies and brains that are breaking down under our current system of health disrupting lifestyle choices. By invoking the changes outlined herein, I have seen many of them improve the quality of their lives immeasurably, even if their commitment is less than 100%. I myself live the 80/20 rule. I allow cheat days, I take rest days. I miss sauna sessions, and ice bath sessions from time to time. No one can be 100% all of the time. I will stress to you, be consistent, and follow the guide 80% of time and reap some great benefits. I do not expect everyone to follow my exact schedule, you will have to find a routine that works for you. Here is what a typical day for me looks like during the week:

- Wake up 5 AM
- 60 minute workout (weights, cardio, circuit training)

- Sit outside with feet in grass, watch sunrise as long as possible (usually 15-20 minutes)
- 3-5 minute ice bath
- Cold shower
- 7AM breakfast
- Work as a Physical Therapist. Try and take lunch between 11 and noon
- 3 PM Supper
- Spend time outside from 4 until sundown. I have three kids in sports, so this is sometimes tougher, sometimes easier depending on season
- 7-9 PM wind down. Turn down lights, wear blue light blocking glasses if we are watching TV, reading, etc.
- 930-10 PM bedtime

Now, I live in Central Illinois, and this schedule changes all of the time. The above schedule is my optimal schedule, but is not the norm. I change my eating window often to suit family and social obligations, I adjust bedtime if we are traveling for sports or activities. I don't always have time for an ice bath or a sauna. I do prioritize morning sun, grounding, blocking blue light at night, keep to an eight hour eating window, sleeping 7-8 hours and exercise daily. Those are non-negotiable for me. The use of a sauna and ice plunge are wonderful and useful, but are bonus tools.

Your next step should be to work on each of the first four chapters as the top priority. Schedule your day around the sunrise and sunset. Get up early, get outside and see the sun with your feet on the ground. Pick your eight hour eating window. Break a sweat with a workout. Once the sun goes down, put on a pair of blue light blocking glasses. Turn off the lights at night and start sleeping soundly for 7-8 hours. Do this everyday, and over the course of the next 30 days you will be a different person. If you can add in a weekly sauna and ice bath, you will accelerate your greatness.

Start your checklist here:

1. See the sunrise
2. Feet in the ground
3. Pick your eight hour eating window
4. Break a sweat
5. Block the blue light at night
6. Embrace the heat and cold

You have the potential to make yourself as healthy as you want to be. Lose weight, feel better, move better and reclaim your life. I see it everyday in the clinic; people overcoming poor choices for decades, and coming back better. Our bodies and minds are designed to take care of themselves, if we just give them the input they desire. I hope this book can be used to get you going in the right direction toward complete independence and freedom from the binds of illness and disability.

Oh, and one final thing that seems to help...get a dog, they make everything better!!

If you found this book helpful, I would truly appreciate a favorable review of the book on Amazon!!

Chapter 7 Resources

7 great reasons why exercise matters. (n.d.). Mayo Clinic. https://www.ma yoclinic.org/healthy-lifestyle/fitness/in-depth/exercise/art-20048389

About chronic diseases. (2024, October 4). Chronic Disease.https://ww w.cdc.gov/chronic-disease/about/index.html

Beabout, L. (2024, October 28). *Circadian Fasting: Benefits, How-TO, and Health Insights.* Greatist. https://greatist.com/health/circadian-rhy thm-fasting#:~:text=Circadian%20rhythm%20fasting%20involves%2 0scheduling,and%20even%20reduce%20destructive%20inflammation .

Cho, Y., Ryu, S., Lee, B. R., Kim, K. H., Lee, E., & Choi, J. (2015). Effects of artificial light at night on human health: A literature review of observational and experimental studies applied to exposure assessment. *Chronobiology International,* 32(9), 1294–1310. https://doi.org/10.3109/0 7420528.2015.1073158

Fischer, K. (2024, May 3). *Grounding: techniques and benefits.* WebMD. https://www.webmd.com/balance/grounding-benefits

Hall, K.-M., RN, BSN, CCRN. (2024, June 21). *8 Ways Sunlight Can Benefit Your Health.* https://www.goodrx.com/. Retrieved November 16, 2024, from https://www.goodrx.com/health-topic/environmental/benefits-of-sunlight

Heart Disease Facts. (2024, October 24). Heart Disease. https://www.cdc.gov/heart-disease/data-research/facts-stats/index.html#:~:text=Heart%20disease%20in%20the%20United%20States&text=Heart%20disease%20is%20the%20leading,every%205%20deaths.12

Jagim, A., Ph. D. (2024, January 30). *Can taking a cold plunge after your workout be beneficial?* https://www.mayoclinichealthsystem.org/hometown-health/speaking-of-health/cold-plunge-after-workouts. Retrieved November 16, 2024, from https://www.mayoclinichealthsystem.org/hometown-health/speaking-of-health/cold-plunge-after-workouts

Johns Hopkins Medicine. (n.d.). *Intermittent Fasting: What is it, and how does it work?* https://www.hopkinsmedicine.org/. Retrieved November 16, 2024, from https://www.hopkinsmedicine.org/health/wellness-and-prevention/intermittent-fasting-what-is-it-and-how-does-it-work https://www.britannica.com/topic/fasting

Kruse, J. (2012a, February 12). *The cold thermogenesis protocol.* Dr. Jack Kruse. https://jackkruse.com/the-evolution-of-the-leptin-rx/

Kruse, J. (2012b, June 3). *Cold Thermogenesis 13: The FAQ's.* Dr. Jack Kruse. https://jackkruse.com/cold-thermogenesis-13-the-faqs/

OBESITY: OVERVIEW OF AN EPIDEMIC. (2012, December 1). https://pmc.ncbi.nlm.nih.gov/articles/PMC3228640/ https://www.niddk.nih.gov/health-information/health-statistics/overweight-obesity. Retrieved November 16, 2024, from https://pmc.ncbi.nlm.nih.gov/articles/PMC3228640/ https://www.niddk.nih.gov/health-information/health-statistics/overweight-obesity

Strength training: Get stronger, leaner, healthier. (n.d.). Mayo Clinic. https://www.mayoclinic.org/healthy-lifestyle/fitness/in-depth/strength-training/art-20046670

What to know about saunas and your health. (2023, September 13).

WebMD. https://www.webmd.com/fitness-exercise/what-to-know-saunas-and-health

About the Author

A little about myself, my name is Joe Fiore and I am a physical therapist with 20+ years of experience in practice and a background in strength and conditioning. I have gone from competitive athlete as a college wrestler to strength and conditioning coach to physical therapist. I have tested all of the techniques in this book on myself and have helped thousands of patients regain function through lifestyle changes and exercise. I have found recently that the ideas and habits outlined in this book have provided the best short term results that turn into long term success for myself and hundreds of patients in my clinic. I truly have a passion for helping others not only recover from injury, but maximize their health for the long haul. I have seen this exact program work time after time from the young athlete trying to enhance performance, to the elderly grandmother taking care of her family. I hope that you can follow through and reach your potential.

www.ingramcontent.com/pod-product-compliance
Lightning Source LLC
Chambersburg PA
CBHW051719250726
48653CB00008B/3101